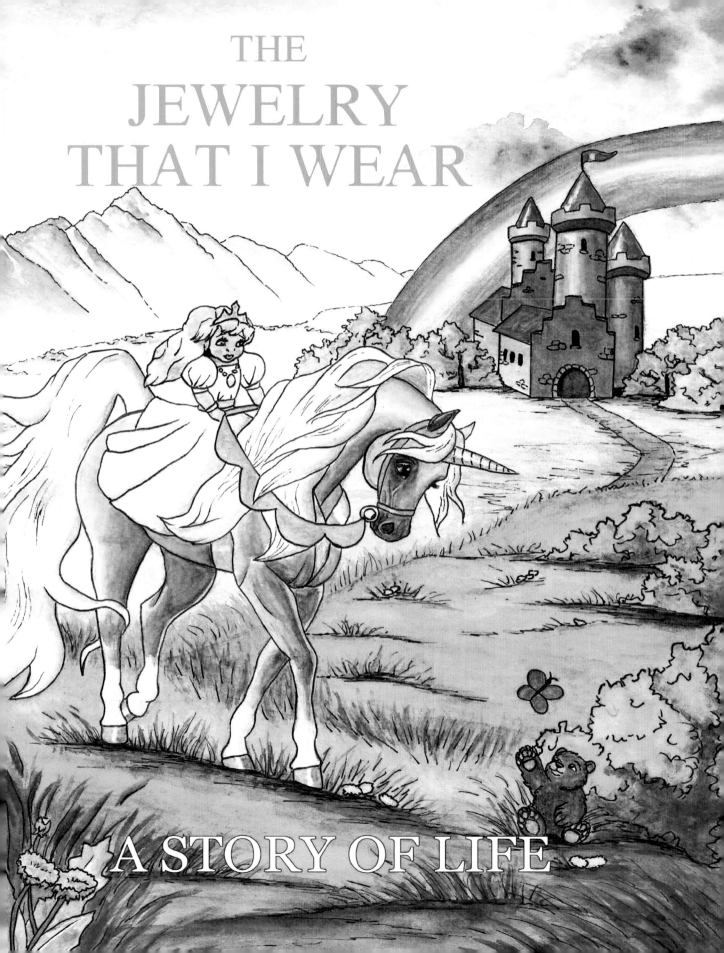

THE JEWELRY THAT I WEAR

A STORY OF LIFE

ISBN: 978-1-938911-68-2

Library of Congress Control Number: 2020909129

Inspired by a True Story

We hope you enjoy this story and the beautiful truths hidden in these pages. The story begins by showing the comforting love of a mother for her child, the simple yet beautiful thoughts of a child, and the princess she becomes as together they dream. A mother's love and compassion for her child has no measure, and they are shown throughout the pages of this story.

May it be a blessing to all those who read it.

I'm just a little girl
Mommy and daddy gave me a little bear

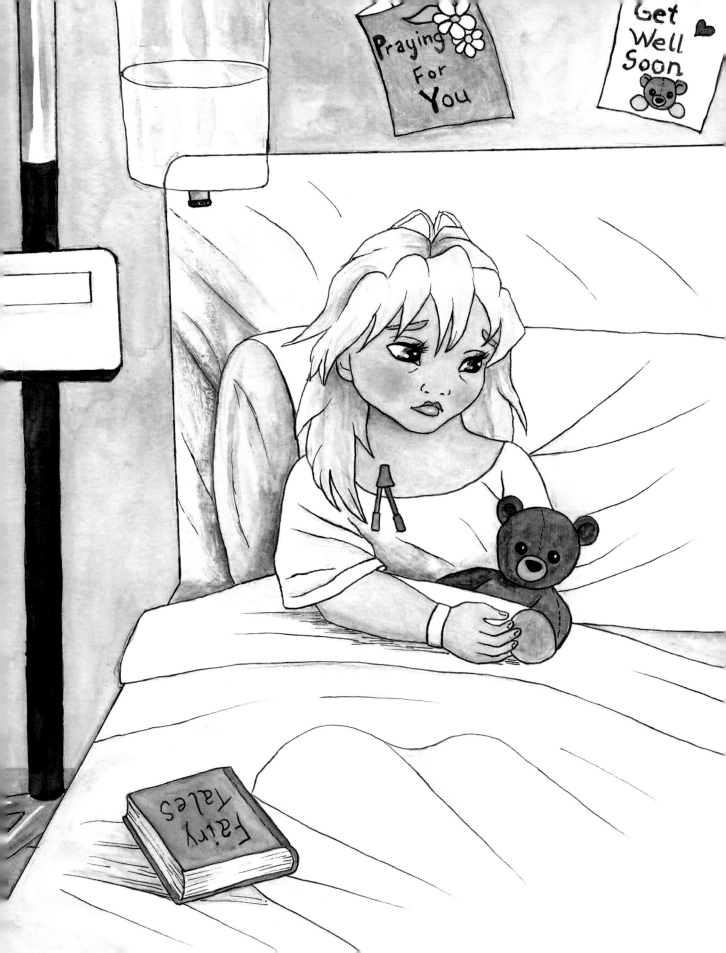

When he looks at me he sees a princess
In the jewelry that I wear

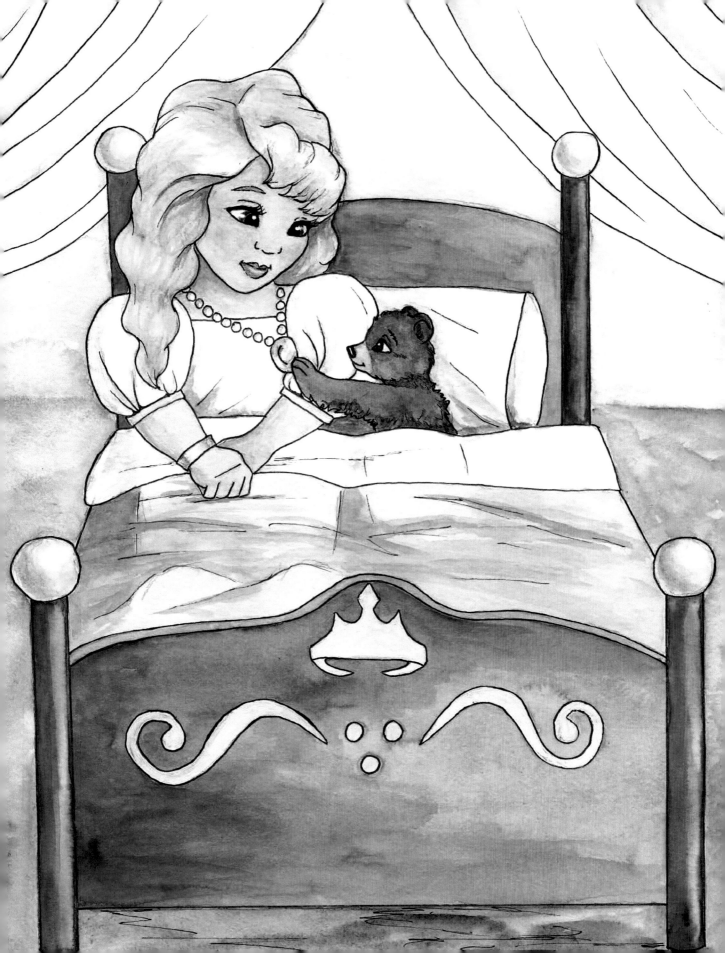

Playing make-believe with mommy
She pretends we haven't got a care

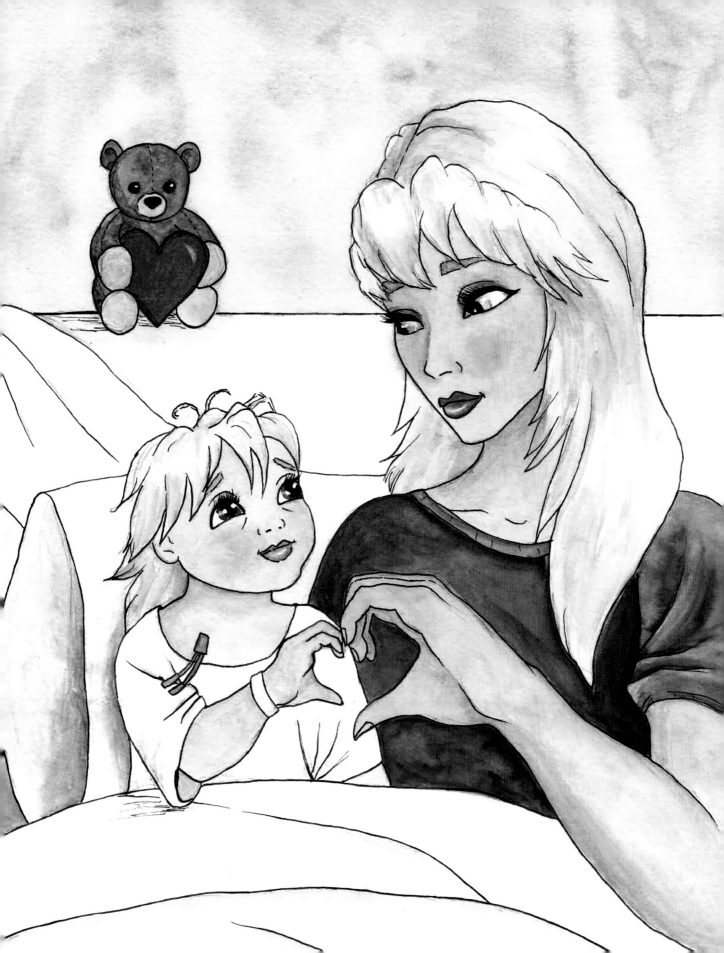

And how I look so pretty
In the jewelry that I wear

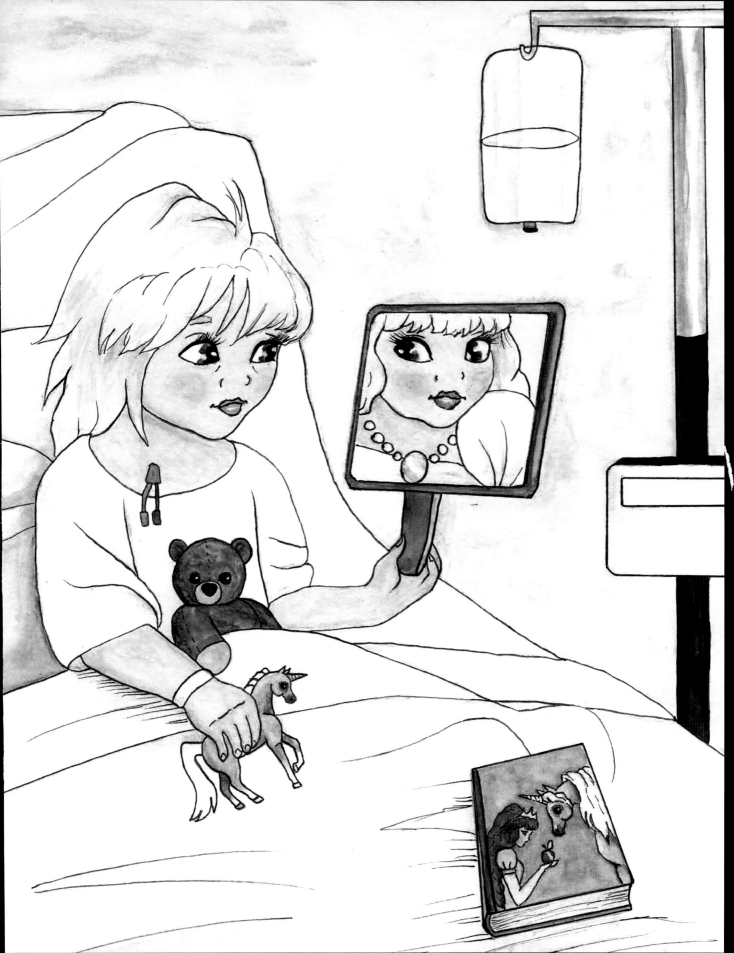

My princess dress is so pretty
White and flowing in the air

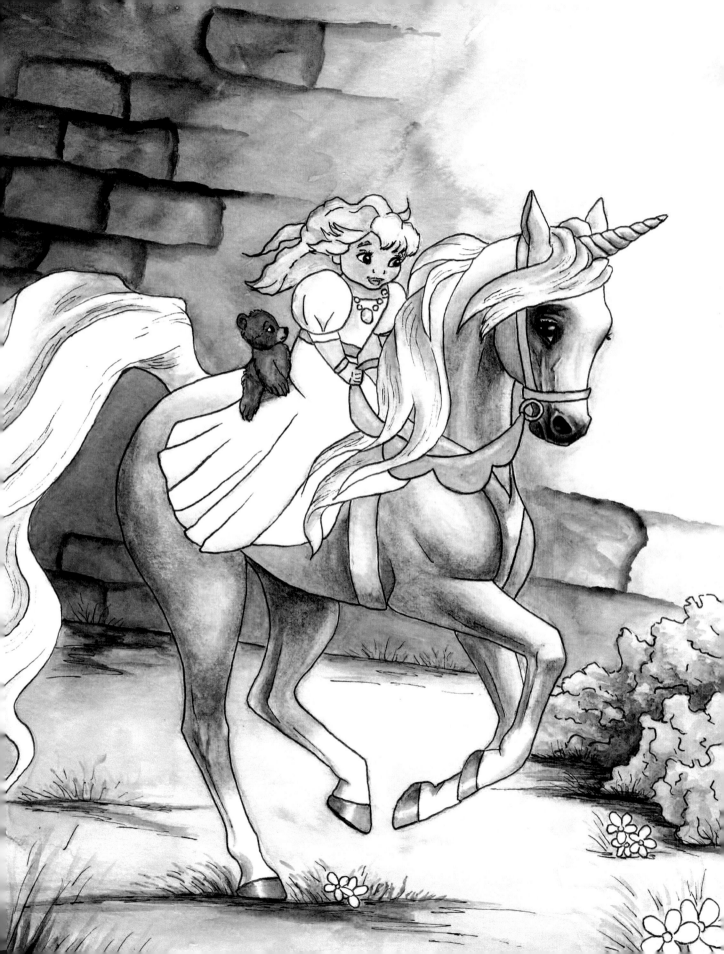

It's on me all the time
Like the jewelry that I wear

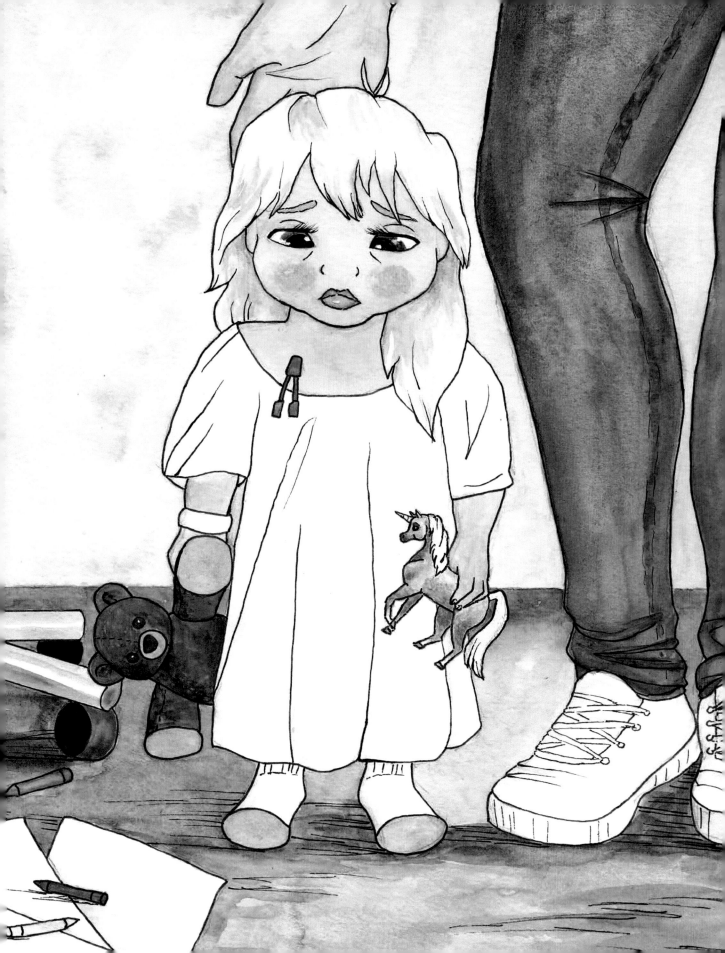

My Crown it is so beautiful
Mommy puts it in my hair

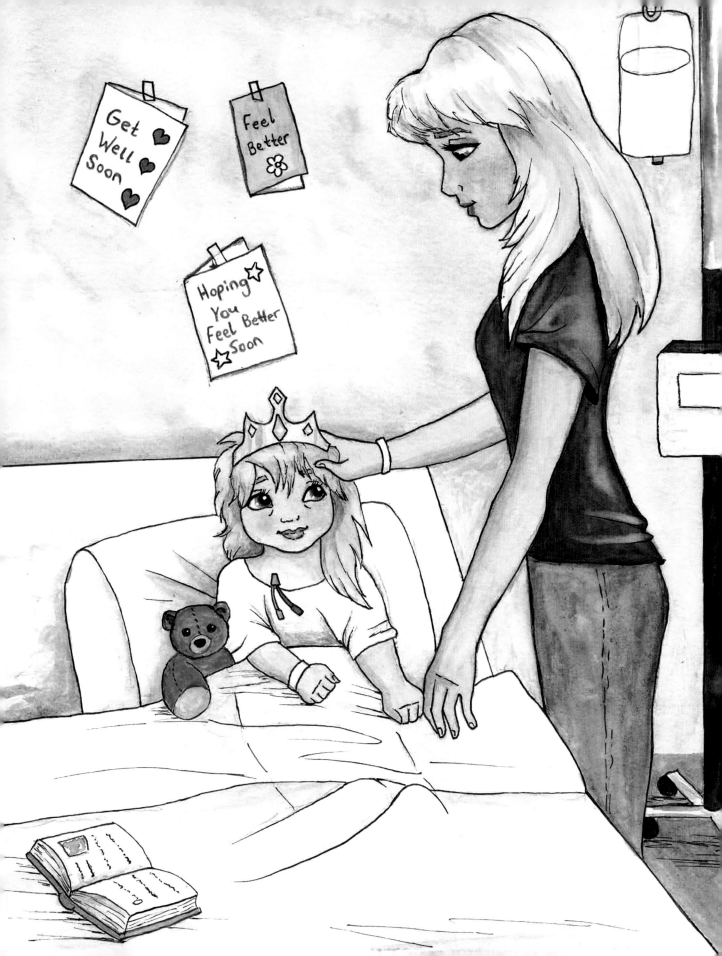

For me it matches perfect
With the jewelry that I wear

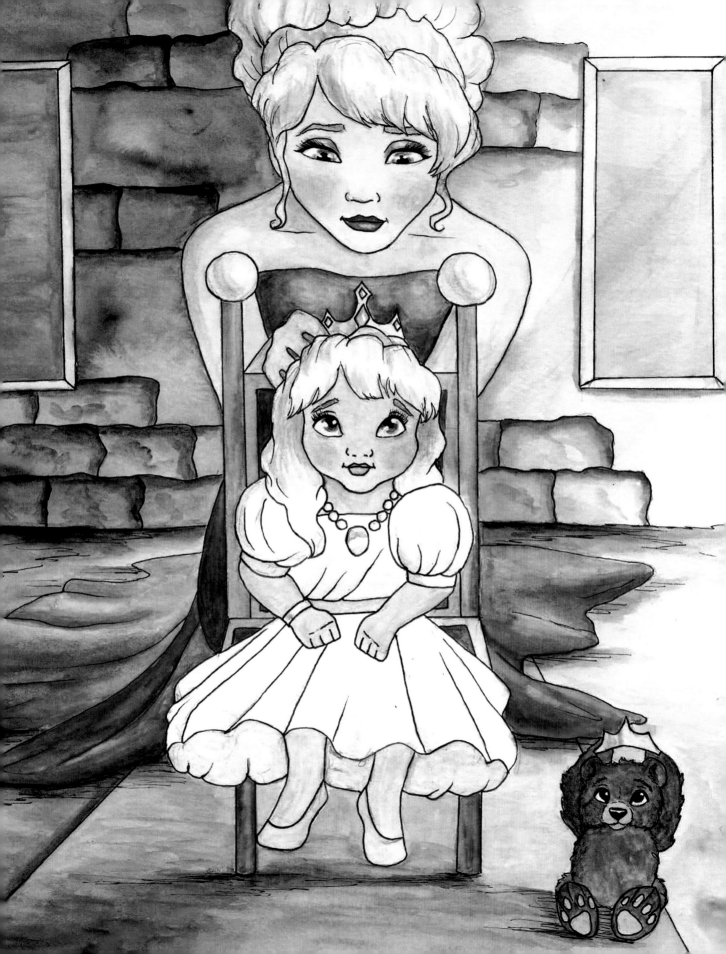

I see my mommy crying
She sits so pretty in her chair

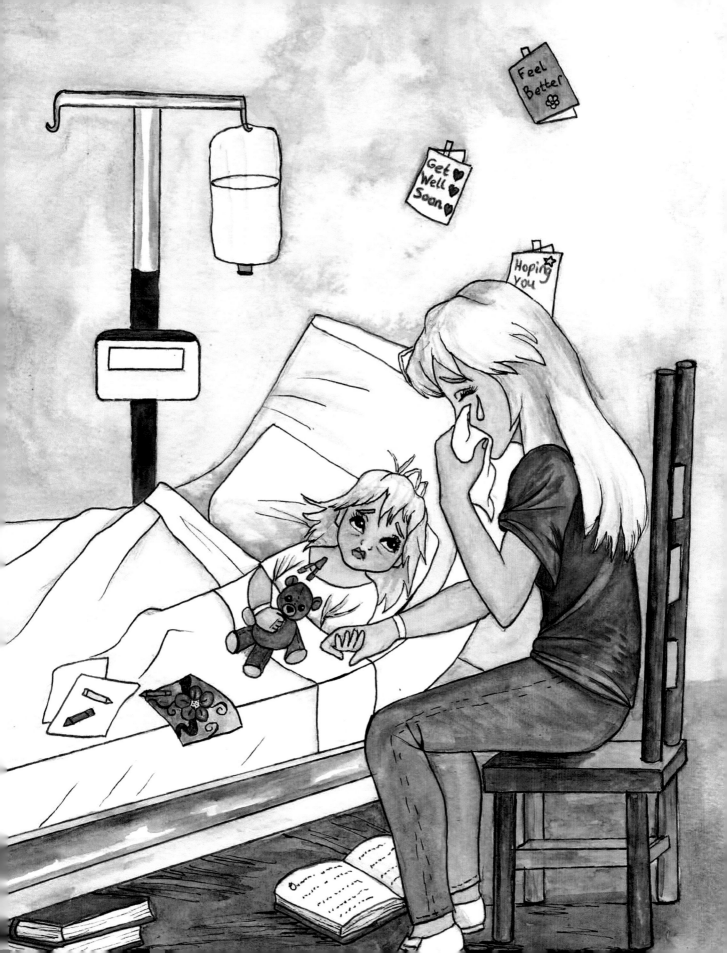

She says that I'm so pretty
In the jewelry that I wear

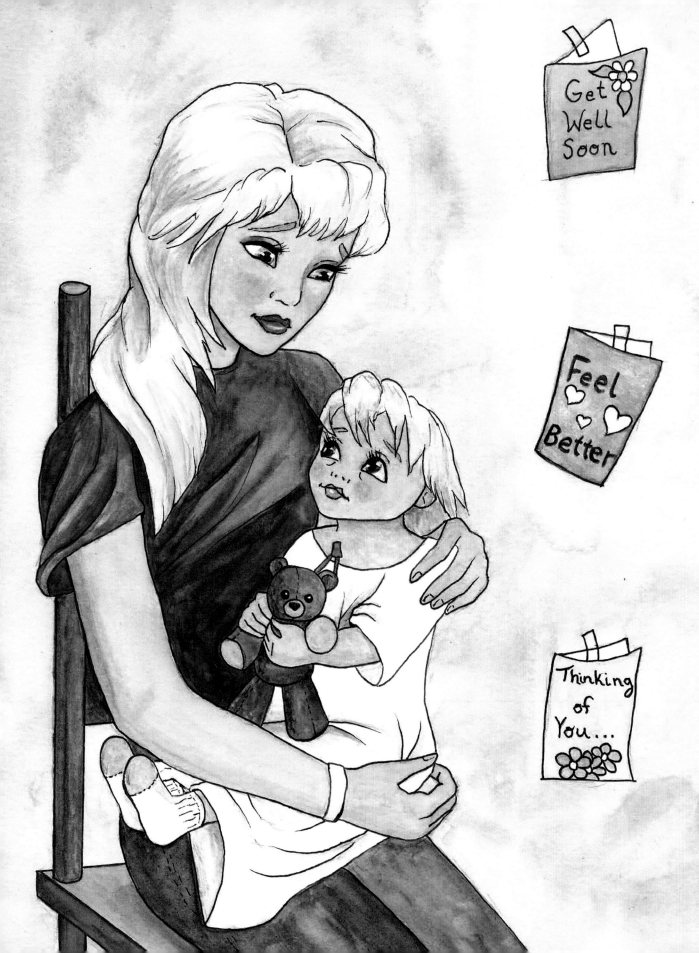

She loves my pretty necklace
She softly cleans it with such care

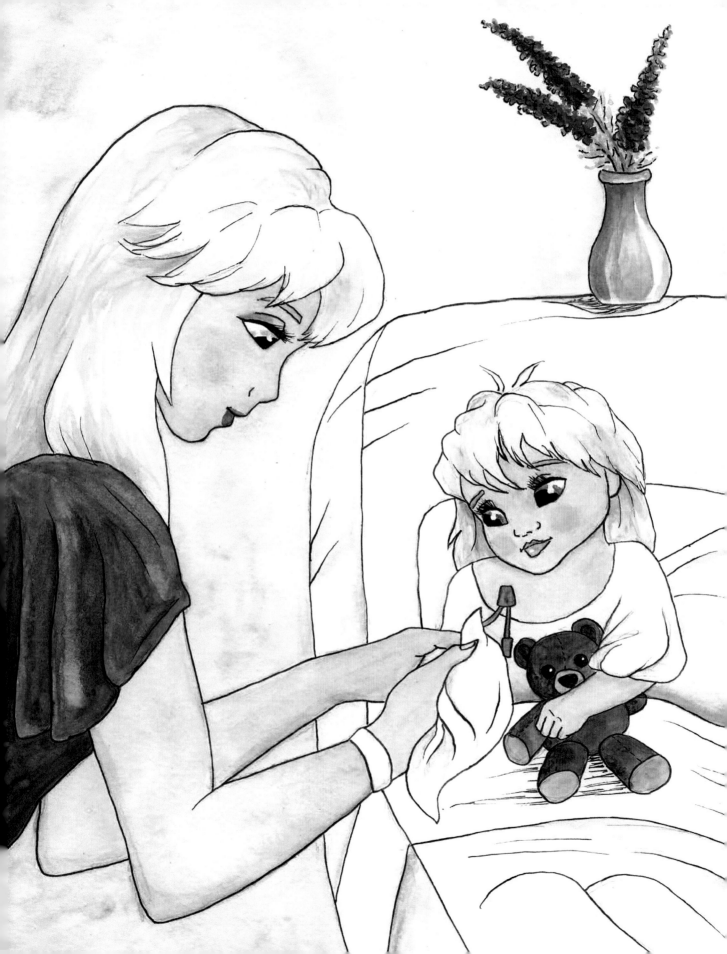

It makes me feel all better
My pretty jewelry that I wear

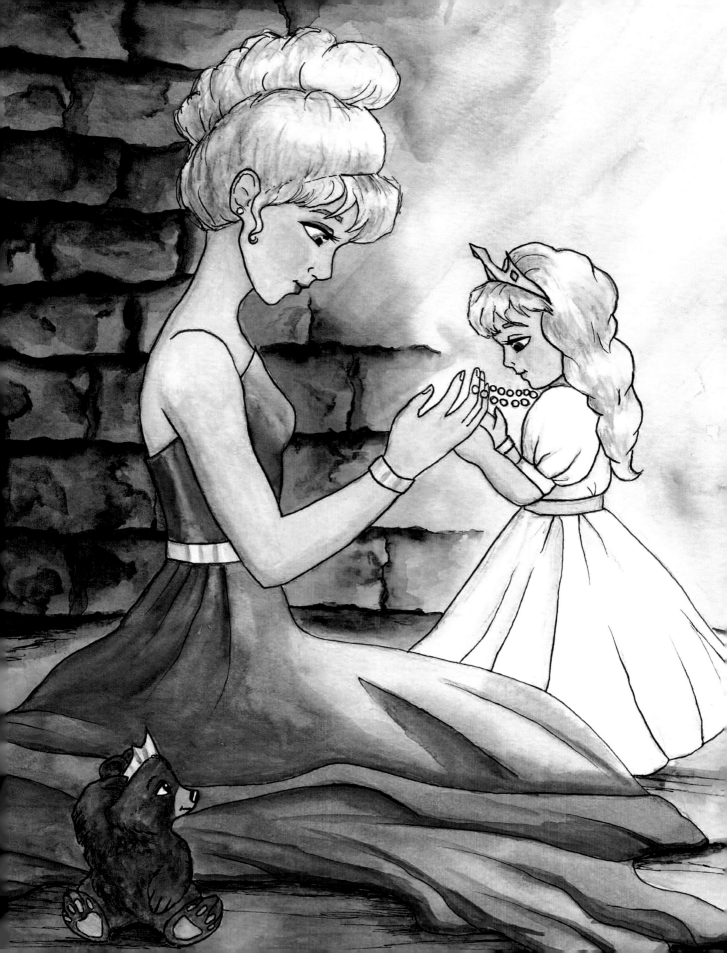

My name is on my bracelet
The name that me and mommy share

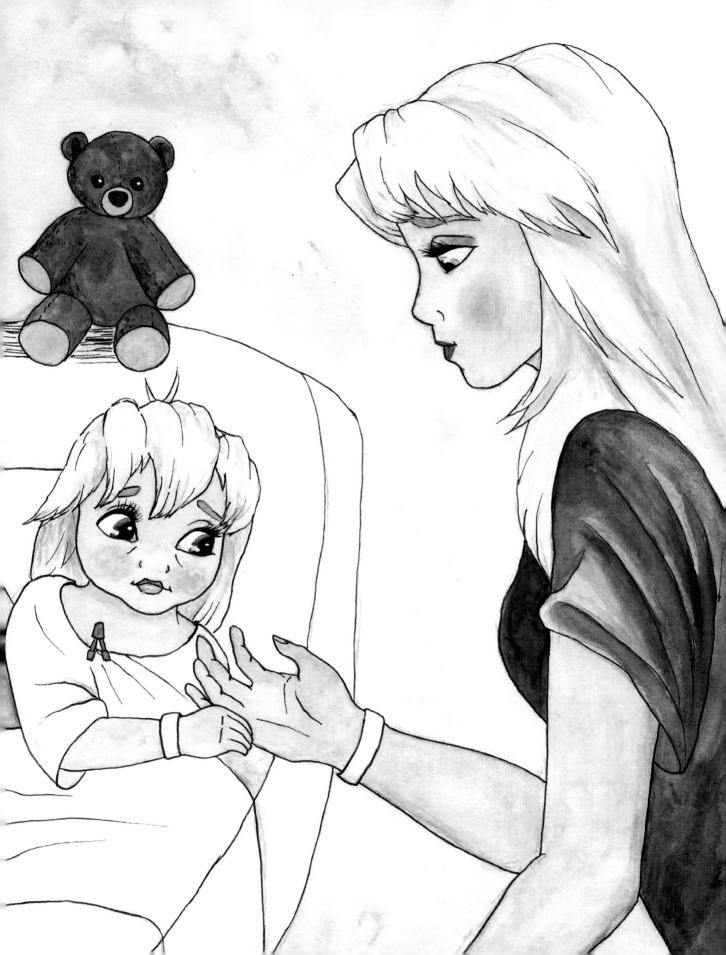

And also with my daddy
On the jewelry that I wear

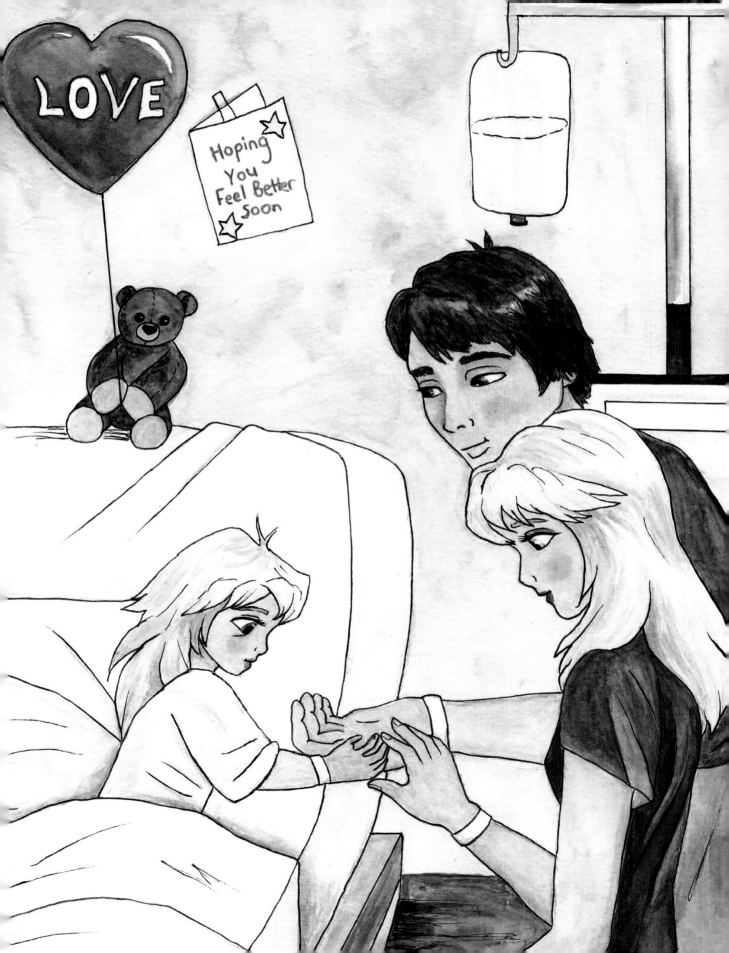

Mommy said someday our Lord Jesus
On Him I will cast all my cares

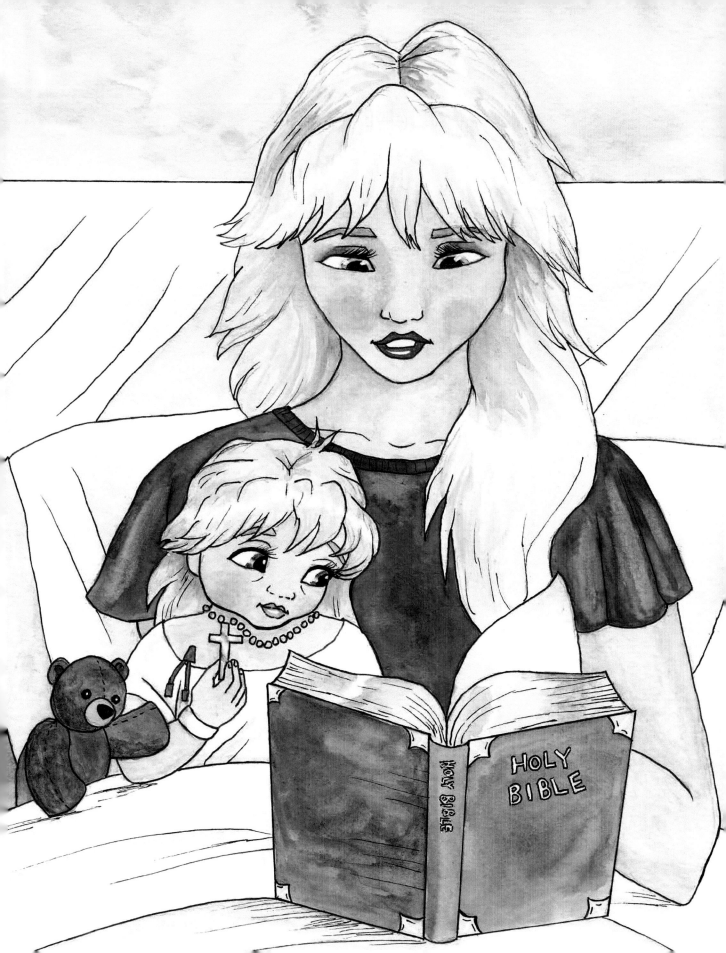

And He will be my jewelry
The jewelry that I wear

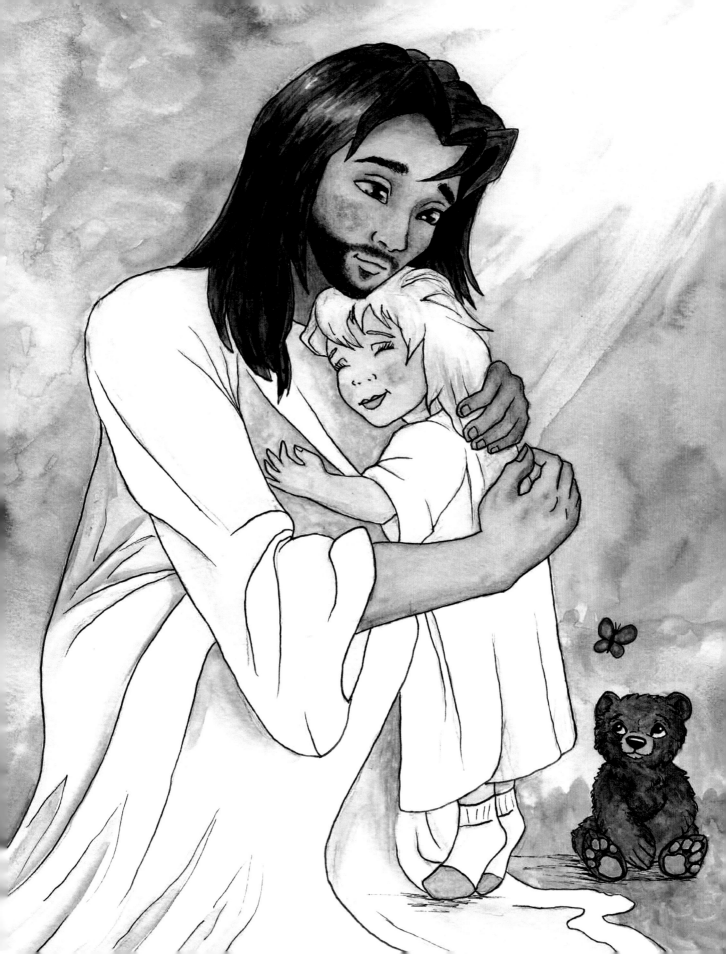

And so they went
Hand in Hand as a family
Enjoying their life together

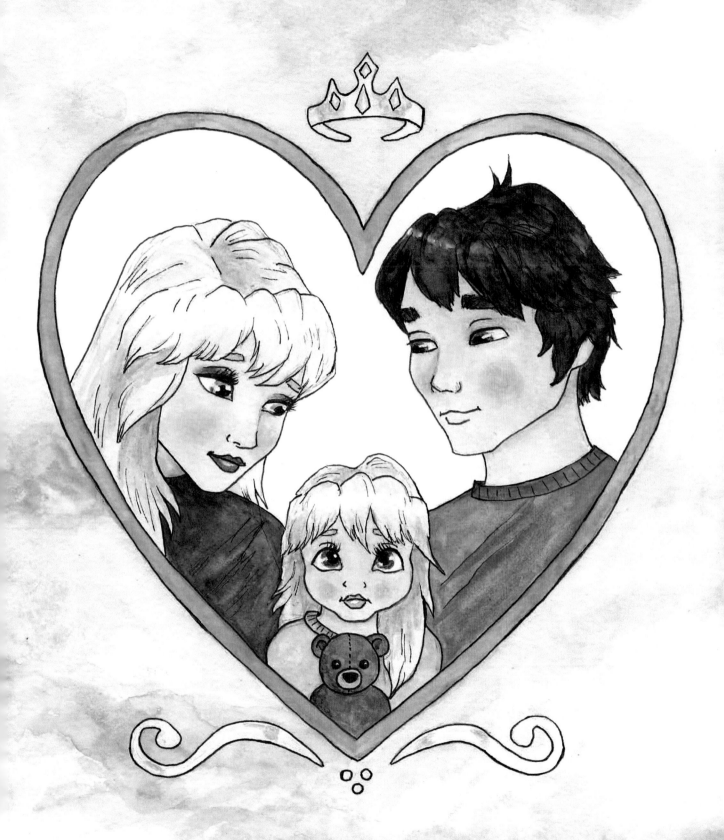

Love is patient, love is kind. It does not envy, it does not boast, it is not proud. It is not rude, it is not self-seeking, it is not easily angered, it keeps no record of wrongs. Love does not delight in evil but rejoices with the truth. It always protects, always trusts, always hopes, always perseveres.